# CHAIR YOGA
# FOR SENIOR OVER 60

*Unlocking vitality, balance, strength, and enhancing life's golden years with just 15 minutes a day*

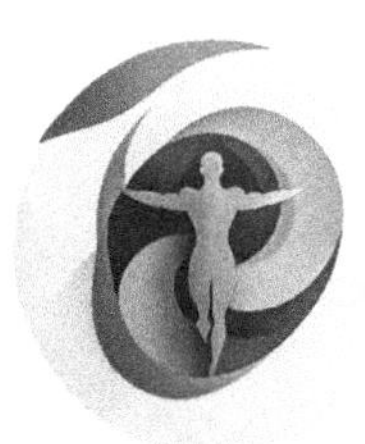

## PRESTON ARIAS

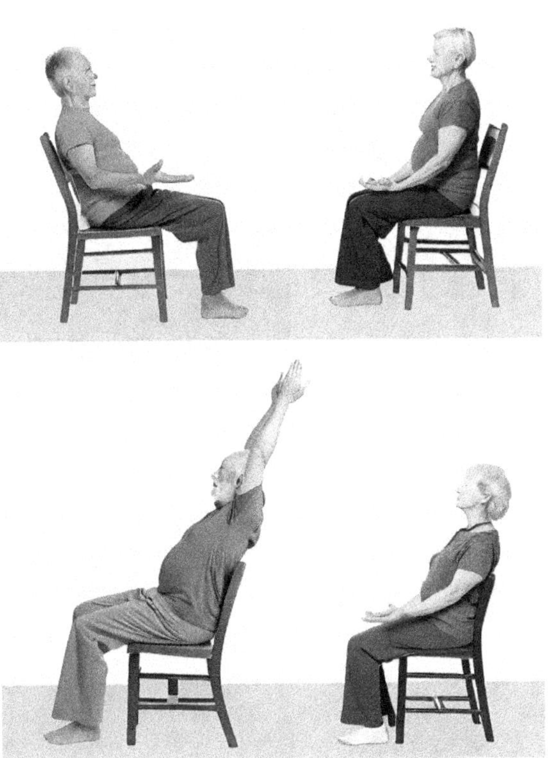

# Dedication

*Dedicated to every senior on a journey to wellness. May this guide to chair yoga be a source of inspiration, strength, and joy as you embrace the golden years with vitality and balance.*

# Table of Contents

# *Author's Note*

**Dear Readers,**

It is with immense gratitude and joy that I present "Chair Yoga for Seniors Over 60." This book is a culmination of my passion for promoting holistic well-being among seniors through the transformative practice of chair yoga.

Having witnessed the profound impact of yoga on individuals' lives, I felt compelled to create a resource specifically tailored to the unique needs and experiences of those navigating the golden years. My hope is that this guide serves as a supportive companion on your journey to vitality, balance, and joy.

I extend my deepest appreciation to every reader who embarks on this path. Your commitment to wellness is an inspiration, and I trust that the insights within these pages will contribute to a life enriched with health, happiness, and a deep connection to your own well-being.

Wishing you a fulfilling and enriching journey through the practice of chair yoga.


**With gratitude,**

**Preston Arias**

# Introduction

## Embracing Wellness in Your Golden Years

Greetings and welcome to "Chair Yoga for Seniors Over 60," where we cordially encourage you to set off on a transforming path towards overall health. It makes sense that as we approach old age, we would look for activities that support our physical and spiritual well-being and help us fully enjoy life. This book delves into the gentle yet potent practice of chair yoga, designed with elders like you in mind.

Chair yoga helps us handle the natural changes that come with aging while still providing a route to health, balance, and joy. Chair yoga helps us develop a sense of inner peace and resilience by strengthening our bodies, calming our thoughts, and practicing accessible postures, mindful breathing, and meditation.

We'll learn about the many advantages of chair yoga for seniors over 60 as we go through the following pages. With topics ranging from increasing strength and flexibility to reducing stress and promoting better sleep, every chapter provides helpful advice and motivation to help you along your health path. Whether you're a novice or an experienced yoga practitioner, this book offers the skills and techniques you need to live well into old age.

So let's go off on this enlightening path of self-discovery, healing, and joyous living—a voyage of chair yoga. Take advantage of this chance to put your health first and make the most of your golden years. You'll find that age is not a barrier to a life of energy, balance, and limitless delight when chair yoga is your partner.

∾

# Chapter One

## Introduction to Chair Yoga

Welcome to the first step in improving your well-being: learning about chair yoga. This chapter will examine the fundamentals of chair yoga as well as its many advantages, especially for seniors sixty years of age and up.

For those with different levels of mobility and fitness, chair yoga provides a gentle yet effective approach to conventional yoga techniques. Chair yoga allows practitioners to experience the transforming power of movement, breath, and mindfulness without the need for complicated or taxing postures through a sequence of sitting and supported positions.

We will explore the fundamentals of chair yoga on these pages, looking at how it develops mental clarity and emotional resilience in addition to physical strength, flexibility, and balance. Chair yoga offers a comprehensive framework for nourishing the body, mind, and soul, ranging from mild stretches to focused breathing exercises.

We'll also address common misunderstandings about chair yoga and explain how it differs from traditional yoga practices as we go on this investigation. You will feel more confident integrating chair yoga into your daily routine and enjoying its benefits if you are aware of its special advantages and flexibility.

Come along with us as we take you on an insightful journey into the core of chair yoga. Together, we'll create the foundation for a practice that will enable you to greet your senior years with vigor, equilibrium, and a revitalized feeling of health.

# What is yoga in a chair?

Chair yoga is a kinder version of yoga that modifies standard postures to be done sitting down or with the assistance of a chair. It is especially made to enable anyone with restricted movement, flexibility, or balance—including seniors over 60—to practice yoga.

Chair yoga is a sequence of adapted yoga postures, stretches, and breathing techniques that are easily executed while sitting on a chair or by utilizing the chair as a prop for stability. In order to support mental, emotional, and physical well-being, the practice places a strong emphasis on conscious breathing, gentle movements, and relaxation methods.

## Advantages of Chair Yoga for Elderly People Over 60

For seniors over sixty, chair yoga is a gentle and accessible technique to practice yoga while seated or using a chair for support. It has several advantages. Here are a few of the main advantages:

**1. Increased flexibility:** Chair yoga uses soft stretches and motions to assist seniors loosen up their muscles and joints without straining their bodies.

**2. Enhanced strength:** Seniors who practice chair yoga can develop and maintain their muscle strength, which is essential for preserving their mobility and balance as they age.

**3. Better posture:** Seniors who practice chair yoga are less likely to have back pain and other musculoskeletal problems because it promotes healthy spine alignment and increases self-awareness.

**4. Increased balance and stability:** Chair yoga helps seniors become more balanced and stable, which can help ward against falls and accidents.

**5. Stress reduction:** Breathing exercises and relaxation methods are incorporated into chair yoga to help relieve stress and enhance mental health in general.

**6. Improved circulation:** The mild stretches and motions of chair yoga can aid in increasing blood flow, which is good for cardiovascular health and may lower the chance of developing diseases like cancer and hypertension.

**7. Enhanced joint mobility:** Seniors with illnesses like arthritis can experience less stiffness and discomfort by maintaining and increasing their range of motion in their joints with the aid of chair yoga.

**8. Enhanced mood:** Because chair yoga emphasizes mindfulness and relaxation and releases endorphins, it can have a mood-boosting impact on practitioners.

**9. Social interaction:** Seniors may engage in the community and socialize with others by taking chair yoga courses, which is beneficial for their general wellbeing.

**10. Accessible exercise option:** Chair yoga is an inclusive and accessible type of exercise that is appropriate for seniors with varying levels of fitness and physical ability.

**11. Enhanced cognitive function:** According to some study, doing yoga, especially chair yoga, may assist older persons' cognitive performance and lower their risk of cognitive decline.

**12. Pain management:** Gentle movement and stretches offered by chair yoga can assist seniors with chronic pain issues feel less uncomfortable and manage their pain more effectively overall.

*For seniors over 60, chair yoga has several advantages that support their mental, emotional, and physical health while encouraging awareness and relaxation.*

# Setting Up Your Practice Space: The First Steps

Establishing a setting that is favorable to chair yoga is crucial to its success. The stages to setting up your practice area are as follows:

**1. Select a Calm Area:** Look for a serene, quiet spot in your house where you can do chair yoga without any interruptions. This might be a spare room, a corner of your living room, or any other area where you feel at ease and content.

**2. Clear the Space:** To make a room that is safe and open for mobility, clear the area of any debris or obstructions. Take away any furniture or other items that might get in the way of your motions while practicing.

**3. Use a robust Chair:** For your practice, choose for a steady, robust chair that isn't on wheels. To avoid the chair tipping over or sliding during the exercise, make sure it is positioned on a level surface.

**4. Adjust the Height:** Make sure you are sitting in a chair that is comfortable for you. With your knees bent at a 90-degree angle, your feet should be flat on the floor. To get the right height, you can, if necessary, place cushions or yoga blocks beneath your feet.

**5. Secure Props :** Assemble any equipment or accouterments that might improve your practice, such straps, yoga blocks, or blankets. Throughout the session, these props might offer extra aid and support.

**6. Create a Calm Environment:** Prepare the space for your exercise by turning down the lights, turning on some soothing music, and, if you'd like, burning candles or incense. Establishing a calm environment might assist you in decompressing and giving your practice your all.

**7. Dress Comfortably:** Don loose, cozy apparel that doesn't restrict your range of motion. Steer clear of constricting apparel that might make it difficult for you to move freely during the session.

**8. Set objectives:** Give your practice a minute to gather its objectives and aims. Whether your goal is to become more flexible, feel less stressed, or just take a time to unwind, being clear about your objectives can help you stay focused and directed during your practice.

*When you carefully arrange your practice area, you create a warm and inviting location where you can truly experience the life-changing powers of chair yoga. When you take the effort to establish a place that promotes and maintains your health, you'll be prepared to start chair yoga with ease and confidence.*

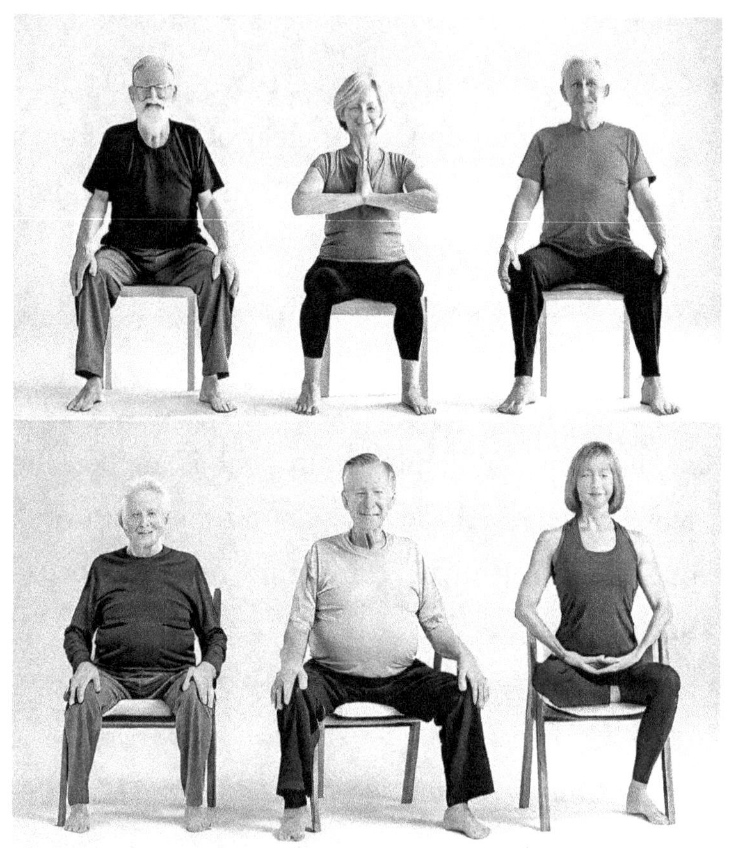

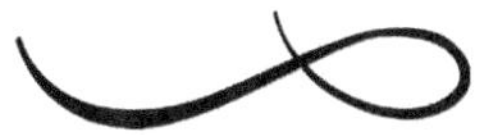

# Chapter Two

# Safety First: Guidelines for Practicing Chair Yoga

When doing chair yoga, safety must always come first, especially for elderly people. We'll go over crucial safety measures and things to think about in this chapter to make the exercise both fun and safe.

## Careful Considerations and Precautions for Seniors

12

**1. Consult Your Healthcare Provider**: It's important to speak with your healthcare provider before beginning any new fitness regimen, including chair yoga, particularly if you have any underlying medical issues or concerns. In addition to providing individualized advice, your healthcare professional can guarantee that chair yoga is suitable for you and safe.

**2. Listen to Your Body:** Throughout the practice, pay special attention to how your body feels. If you feel any pain, discomfort, or lightheadedness, stop right away and adjust or skip the posture as necessary. Recognize the limits of your body and refrain from going beyond your comfort zone.

**3. Use Props for Support:** To offer extra stability and support to your practice, use props like yoga blocks, blankets, or cushions. Props can lower your chance of injury and assist you maintain correct alignment, particularly if you have restricted mobility or flexibility.

**4. Avoid Overexertion:** Take it slow and try not to push yourself too hard, particularly if you're new to chair yoga or haven't worked out in a while. As your strength and endurance build, start out slowly and progressively increase the time and intensity of your practice.

**5. Modify Poses as Needed:** Be open to changing positions to accommodate your unique requirements and skill level. Not every position is appropriate for every person, therefore it's critical to identify modifications or substitutes that best suit your body. Any physical restrictions or difficulties can be accommodated by you by modifying postures with the assistance of your instructor or a trained yoga teacher.

**6. Remain Hydrated:** To keep hydrated and replace fluids lost via perspiration, drink lots of water prior to, during, and after your chair yoga exercise. Keep drinking water during your practice since dehydration can worsen muscle fatigue and raise the chance of injury.

**7. Cultivate Mindful Awareness:** Throughout your practice, pay attention to your breath, your body's sensations, and your thoughts. During the practice, mindfulness can help you avoid mishaps or injuries, stay in the present time, and minimize distractions.

*You may minimize the danger of pain or damage while still reaping the many advantages of chair yoga by taking some safety measures and considerations. Always put safety first. A safe and fulfilling chair yoga practice depends on respecting your body's requirements and limits.*

# Adjustments and Attachments for Suitability and Comfort

For seniors in particular, adjustments and props are essential to guaranteeing comfort and support during chair yoga sessions. Here are a few typical adjustments and accessories you can utilize:

**1. Chair Modifications:** Experiment with different chair postures to see what works best for you. For instance, you can bend your knees or lay a cushion on your thighs for support if a sitting forward bend feels too difficult.

**2. Use of Props:** During postures, props like yoga blocks, blankets, or straps can offer extra help and support. For example, a strap can assist you reach your feet while bending forward while seated, and blankets can offer additional padding for joints that are particularly uncomfortable.

**3. Adjusting Seat Height:** To guarantee correct alignment and comfort, place cushions or yoga blocks beneath your feet if your chair is too high or too low for a certain posture.

**4. Wall Support:** You can utilize a nearby wall or a solid piece of furniture for stability and support as you practice standing postures or balancing exercises.

**5. Chair Back Support:** If you find it difficult to sit still for long periods of time, you might want to choose a chair with a backrest that supports your lower back or place a cushion behind your lower back for more comfort.

# Paying Attention to Your Form: Engaging in Mindful Awareness

A key component of chair yoga is mindful awareness, which enables you to develop a closer relationship with your body and prevent injury or overexertion. The following advice can help you cultivate attentive awareness:

**1. Tune into Sensations:** During each stance, become aware of the sensations in your body. To prevent strain, pay attention to any places that are tight, uncomfortable, or tense and modify your motions accordingly.

**2. Inhale Mindfully:** Ground your consciousness in the here and now by using your breath as a guide. As you progress through each posture, pay attention to the rhythm of your breath and let it come to you freely.

**3. Stay Present:** Focus entirely on the here and now, letting go of anxieties and distractions. As you practice, use all of your senses, paying attention to the sights, sounds, and sensations around you without passing judgment.

**4. Modify as Needed:** To ensure comfort and safety, pay attention to your body's cues and adjust positions as necessary. Keep in mind that there is no one-size-fits-all method when it comes to yoga, and it's OK to modify the poses to match your particular requirements and skill level.

*You may create a secure, encouraging, and profoundly nourishing practice for your body, mind, and spirit in chair yoga by utilizing modifications, props, and conscious awareness. As you discover how chair yoga may alter your life, don't forget to respect your body's wisdom and pay attention to its indications.*

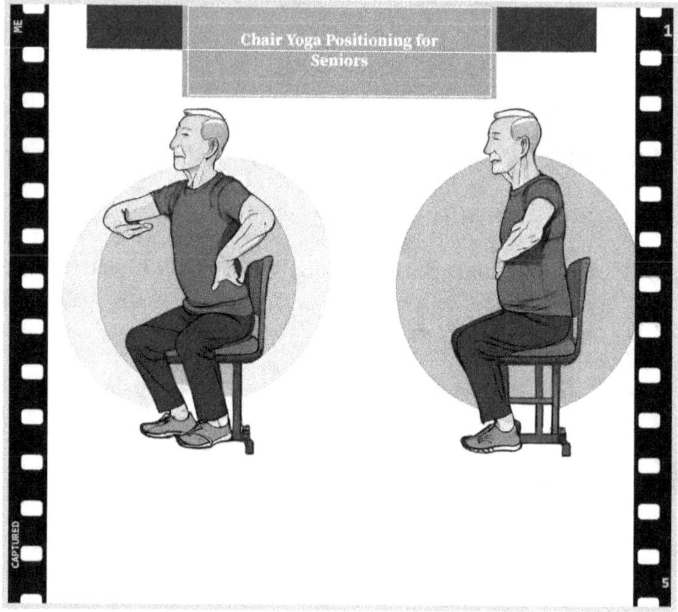

Chair Yoga Positioning for Seniors

# Chapter Three

# Fundamental Chair Yoga Positions and Exercises

We will look at a number of fundamental chair yoga postures and exercises in this chapter that will help you become more flexible, strong, and calm. These mild workouts are designed especially for adults over 60 and provide a convenient and safe means to enhance mobility and general health.

# Warm-Up Stretches to Increase Flexibility

**1. Neck Rolls:** Take a comfortable seat on your chair with your feet flat on the ground and your spine straight. Gently bring your chin up to your chest and spin your head back and forth, letting each ear come close to your shoulder. Repeat many times, taking your time and being conscious.

**2. Shoulder Rolls:** Feel a light stretch over your chest and upper back as you inhale as you raise your shoulders toward your ears and exhale as you roll them back down. Several times over, repeat this action while synchronizing your breathing.

**3. Seated Forward Bend:** Place your feet flat on the floor and sit closer to the edge of your chair. Breathe in as you extend your back and out as you bend forward from your hips and reach for your shins or feet. Retain a flat back and refrain from bending your spine. After a few breaths, hold the stretch, and then carefully come back up to your normal posture.

**4. Seated Side Stretch:** Take a tall seat on your chair and make sure your feet are firmly planted on the ground. Sensation stretches down the left side of your body when you raise your left arm aloft and tilt slightly to the right. After holding for a few breaths, alternate sides and perform the exercise on the other.

**5. Seated Spinal Twist:** Place your feet firmly on the floor and sit toward the front of your chair. Put your left hand on the chair's back and your right hand on the outside of your left knee. Breathe in to extend your spine; when you gaze over your left shoulder and twist slightly to the left, release the breath. After a few breaths, hold the twist, then come back to the center and repeat on the opposite side.

*This mild warm-up is a great way to get your body ready for more challenging chair yoga postures and exercises. Regular practice will increase your range of motion, lessen stiffness, and encourage calmness and wellbeing in your day-to-day activities.*

# Exercises to Build Strength and Vitality

**1. Chair Squats:** To start, place your feet hip-width apart and sit toward the front of your chair. Using the strength in your legs, steadily rise up by utilizing your core. With control, lower yourself back into the chair. To increase the strength in your lower body, repeat numerous times.

**2. Leg Lifts:** Place your feet flat on the floor and sit tall in your chair. Using your thigh muscles, extend one leg straight out in front of you and then raise it a few inches off the ground. After a little period of time, release your leg. Continue on the opposite side. This workout increases leg strength and strengthens the quadriceps.

**3. Seated Row:** with your feet flat on the floor and a resistance band looped around your feet, assume a seated row position. With your palms facing each other, grasp one end of the resistance band in each hand. Press the band in the direction of your chest while bringing your shoulder blades together. Return to the starting position slowly. This exercise helps with posture and develops the upper back muscles.

*Adding these strengthening poses to your chair yoga practice can help you achieve better muscular tone, more energy, and better physical health overall. As your strength and confidence grow, gradually increase from a few repetitions to a larger number.*

# Poses Balanced for Confidence and Stability

**1. One-Leg Balance:** Take a tall seat on your chair, raise one foot off the floor, and balance on the other. If necessary, use the chair's back as support. To assist in keeping your body stable, contract your core muscles. Take a few breaths to maintain the equilibrium, then swap sides. This workout develops the muscles in the legs and core and enhances balance.

**2. Sitting Tree Pose Variation:** Lie on your back with your feet flat on the ground. Taking a comfortable posture, place your right foot on the inner of your left thigh or leg. Put your hands together, palms to palms, at the center of your heart. To aid with balance, contract your core and concentrate on an object in front of you. After a few breaths of holding, switch sides. This position improves focus and steadiness.

**3. Seated Eagle Arms:** Take a lofty seat in your chair and raise your arms to shoulder level. Bending at the elbows, cross your right arm over your left, then round each other with your forearms, bringing your palms together if you can. Raise your elbows a little and extend your back to your shoulder blades. After a few breaths of holding, release and swap sides. Balance, posture, and upper body strength are all enhanced by this stance.

**4. Chair Warrior III:** Place your feet hip-width apart and sit closer to the front of the chair. Raise your arms shoulder-high in front of you. Raise your right leg straight back behind you while simultaneously extending your arms forward by using your core and hunching forward from your hips. Maintain a flat back and level hips. After a few breaths of holding, switch sides and stand back up. This position tests your equilibrium while building stronger upper body, core, and leg muscles.

**5. Half Moon Pose:** Sit upright, placing your feet level on the ground and keeping your arms by your sides. Breathe in as you extend your right arm across your side of the body and upward toward the ceiling. Breathe out and sag slightly to the left while maintaining a planted right hip on the chair. After a few breaths of holding, move back to the middle and repeat on the opposite side. This position increases confidence, expands the side body, and enhances balance.

# Relaxation Methods for Reduction of Stress and Rejuvenation

**1. Deep Breathing:** Take a comfortable seat in your chair, place your hands on your thighs and your feet flat on the ground. Shut your eyes and inhale deeply through your nose, letting your belly swell to its utmost capacity. After holding your breath for a little while, release all of your tension and stress with each leisurely breath out of your lips. For many minutes, keep up this deep breathing exercise while paying attention to how your breath enters and exits your body.

**2. Progressive Muscle Relaxation:** Tense your toes and feet as much as you can, then gradually let go of the tension so that your muscles may relax fully. Tension each muscle area for a few seconds before releasing it; start with your calves and work your way up to your thighs, belly, chest, arms, and lastly, your face and neck. This method encourages profound relaxation throughout the body and aids in the release of physical stress.

**3. Visualization:** Shut your eyes and visualize yourself in a calm and pleasant setting, such a lovely beach, verdant forest, or snug mountain lodge. Allow yourself to completely immerse yourself in the experience by using all of your senses to vividly visualize the sights, sounds, scents, and sensations of this tranquil environment. In addition to lowering tension and fostering a sense of inner serenity and wellbeing, visualization can assist the mind.

**4. Mindful Awareness:** Focus on your breathing, your body's sensations, and your environment without passing judgment in order to bring your attention to the here and now. Take note of the noises and odors in your surroundings, the rise and fall of your chest with each breath, and the feel of the air against your skin. Cultivate a sense of peace and presence by allowing yourself to completely enjoy the present moment without being sucked into worry or other distractions.

**5. Guided Imagery:** Play a guided meditation or relaxation tape that walks you through a sequence of peaceful visualizations and breathing techniques. Guided imagery sessions are offered by several applications, websites, and online platforms with a focus on relaxation and stress management. Let go of any stress and allow your thoughts to wander into a state of profound relaxation and rejuvenation as you follow the instructions.

*By adding these relaxation methods to your chair yoga practice, you may improve your general well-being, ease stress, and encourage a sense of peace and rejuvenation. To promote your mental and emotional well-being, try out several strategies until you find the ones that work best for you. You should also schedule regular time for self-care and relaxation.*

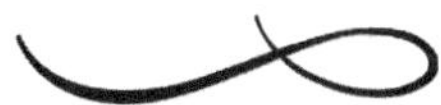

# Chapter Four

# Meditation and Breathing Techniques

We'll look at the tremendous effects of breathing exercises and meditation on your mental, emotional, and physical health in this chapter. You may develop a sense of calm, clarity, and inner peace by practicing mindfulness meditation and pranayama (breath control) practices.

**The Breath's Power:** Utilizing Pranayama Methods to Promote Calm and Clarity

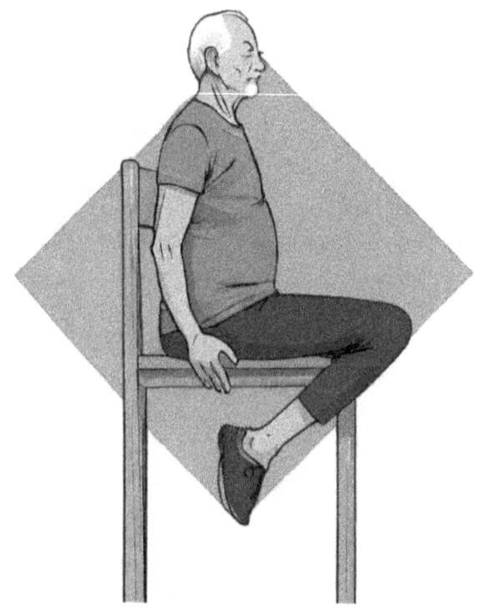

**1. Deep Belly Breathing (Diaphragmatic Breathing):** Take a comfortable chair seat, place your hands on your abdomen, and keep your feet flat on the ground. Inhale deeply through your nose, filling your lungs with air while you let your belly grow to its fullest. To fully empty your lungs, exhale softly via your lips while bringing your belly to your spine. For many minutes, repeat this deep belly breathing rhythm, paying attention to the rise and fall of your abdomen with each breath. This method aids in triggering the body's relaxation response, which lowers tension and fosters serenity.

**2. Original Nostril Breathing (Nadi Shodhana):** Assume a comfortable sitting position, keeping your back straight and placing your left hand on your left knee. Breathe deeply through your left nostril while closing your right nostril with your thumb. Next, gently exhale through your right nostril while closing your left nostril with your right ring finger. Take a breath via your right nostril, shut it with your fingers, then release the breath through your left nostril. For several rounds, keep up this alternate pattern while concentrating on your breath's steady, fluid rhythm. Nadi Shodhana facilitates calmness and relaxation by balancing the body's energy flow.

**3. deep Breath (Victorious Breath):** Close your eyes and sit comfortably with a tall spine. Take a deep breath through your nose and gently tighten the back of your throat to produce a sound that sounds like ocean waves—as when you fog up a mirror. Breathe out gently through your nostrils while keeping your throat constricted to create the same audible sound. For a few minutes, keep doing this ujjayi breath, letting the repetitive sound center your attention and soothe your thoughts. Ujjayi breath lowers stress and increases mental clarity and attention by regulating the neurological system.

*You may use the breath to create a sense of calm, clarity, and inner peace by using these pranayama methods into your chair yoga practice. To feel the profound effects of breath work on your general well-being, practice on a regular basis.*

# Mindfulness-Based Stress Reduction for Inner Calm and Wellness

The technique of mindfulness meditation entails directing your deliberate attention into the current moment, judgment-free. It is possible to develop a stronger sense of inner calm, clarity, and wellbeing via mindfulness meditation. This is how to begin:

**1. Assemble in a Cozy Position:** Locate a peaceful, cozy spot to sit on your chair, placing your hands softly on your lap or thighs and your feet flat on the ground. Whichever way makes you feel most comfortable, close your eyes or avert your attention.

**2. Pay Attention to Your Breath:** Start by focusing on your breathing. As you breathe normally, pay attention to how each inhalation and exhalation feels. You can concentrate on how your belly rises and falls or how your nostrils feel as air enters and exits.

**3. Observe Your Thoughts :** While you keep breathing, you could become aware of ideas coming to mind. Rather than allowing these ideas to consume you or suppress them, just watch them with curiosity and without passing judgment. Visualize your thoughts as fleeting clouds drifting past overhead.

**4. Return to the current Moment:** Focus on your breathing to gently bring your attention back to the current moment whenever you see it straying. To help you return to the present moment, you may also utilize a basic anchor, such as how your body feels in the chair or the sounds that are all around you.

**5. Practice Non-Judgmental Awareness:** Develop a non-judgmental attitude toward your experiences throughout your meditation. Rather than attempting to alter or oppose the ideas, feelings, or sensations that come, accept them. Give yourself permission to just be in the now with whatever is there.

**6. Conclude with Gratitude:** As your meditation draws to a close, spend a few moments thinking about the blessings in your life. This might be anything from little happy experiences to family support. Gratitude cultivation can assist in changing your viewpoint to one that is happier and more optimistic.

# Building Joy and Gratitude: Heart-Centered Exercises

Developing joy and practicing thankfulness are two effective strategies to take care of your heart and improve your general wellbeing. The following are some heart-centered routines you can adopt:

**1. Gratitude Diary:** Assign a certain time each day to jot down three things for which you are thankful. These might be small joys, kind deeds, or breathtaking experiences you've encountered all day long. By focusing on the positive aspects of your life, you may develop a sense of plenty and gratitude while diverting your attention from negativity.

**2. Random Acts of compassion:** Seek for chances to show compassion to others. This can take the shape of a smile, a sympathetic ear, or a tiny deed of service. Kindness not only helps others but also makes your own life happier and more fulfilling.

**3. Mindful Appreciation:** Set aside some time each day to focus on the wonder and beauty of the environment you live in. Take note of the flavors of your favorite dish, the hues of the sky at sunrise, or the sound of chirping in the morning. Discovering delight and amazement in everyday experiences can be facilitated by practicing mindful gratitude.

**4. Meditation with Loving Kindness:** Engage in a loving-kindness meditation in which you send blessings of health, happiness, and tranquility to both yourself and other people. Start silently repeating affirmations like "May I be happy, may I be healthy, may I be at peace," and then progressively include family, friends, and even people you may not get along with in your wishes. Developing empathy and kindness for both yourself and other people can provide a stronger sense of connectedness and wellbeing.

*You may create a deeper feeling of inner peace, pleasure, and well-being by implementing heart-centered activities,* mindfulness meditation, and gratitude practices into your everyday life. These practices provide us with strong skills to help us face life's obstacles head-on and bounce back, as well as to help us cherish the fleeting moments of happiness and connection that make life worthwhile.

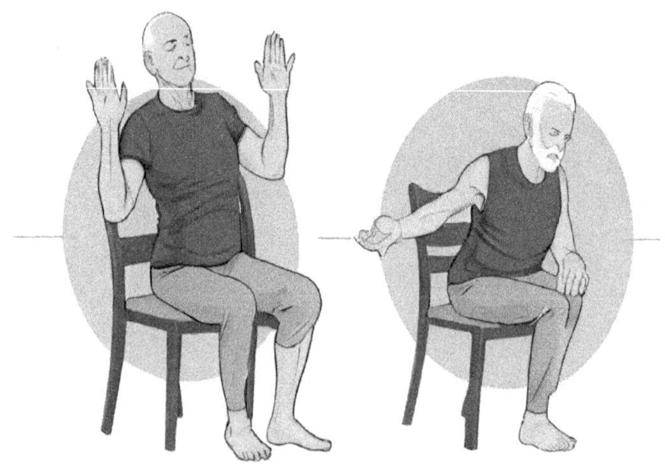

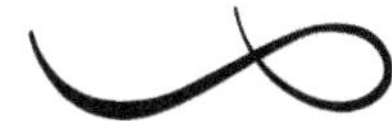

# Chapter Five

# Incorporating Chair Yoga into Daily Life

This chapter will discuss how to include chair yoga into your regular practice to reap all of its advantages and improve your general health.

# Creating a Consistent Practice Schedule

**1. Set Realistic Goals:** To begin with, decide what you want to get out of your chair yoga practice. Think on how many times a week you would want to practice and how long each session will last. As your consistency and confidence grow, start with little objectives like practicing three times a week for fifteen minutes each, and then progressively expand.

**2. Select a Convenient Time:** To add chair yoga into your routine, decide on a time of day that works best for you. Select a time when you are most likely to maintain your practice regularly, such as first thing in the morning to invigorate your day, during a lunch break to refresh and recharge, or in the evening to unwind and relax.

**3. Set Up a Dedicated Space:** Choose a room in your house where you can comfortably and noise-free do chair yoga. Make the area welcoming, clutter-free, and supportive of mindfulness and relaxation. Maintaining a regular practice will be simpler if you have a designated area.

**4. Start Small:** Practice for shorter periods of time at first if you're new to chair yoga or have a hectic schedule. As you gain comfort and confidence, you can practice for longer periods of time. Chair yoga, even for ten to fifteen minutes a day, may have a profound impact on your physical and emotional health.

**5. Be Adaptive and adaptable:** Since life is unpredictable, adjust and be adaptable in how you approach your exercise regimen. Try not to be too harsh on yourself if you skip a scheduled session. Alternatively, look for creative ways to include chair yoga into your day, including doing a few light stretches while watching TV or pausing during the workday to take a mindful breathing exercise.

**6. Set Accountability and Reminders:** To help you remember to frequently practice chair yoga, set alarms, reminders, or calendar notifications. A friend, relative, or online group can also help you by holding you responsible and offering encouragement as you go.

**7. Celebrate Your Progress:** As you advance in chair yoga, acknowledge and appreciate your accomplishments. Recognize and appreciate the beneficial effects of your practice on your general well-being, whether it be increased flexibility, a sense of calm and centering, or just finding time for self-care in the middle of a hectic schedule.

**8. Above all,** pay attention to what your body is telling you and respect its boundaries. Give yourself permission to take a break day or adjust your practice as necessary if you're feeling worn out or ill. Chair yoga is all about taking care of your body, mind, and soul, so put your health and wellbeing first.

*You may reap the life-changing advantages of chair yoga by making it a regular practice and incorporating it into your daily routine. Chair yoga is a moderate and accessible type of exercise. Since consistency is essential, resolve to incorporate chair yoga into your self-care regimen on a regular basis and reap the benefits it provides for your mental, emotional, and physical well-being.*

# Customizing Your Methods to Meet Particular Requirements or Issues

**1. Assess Your Needs:** To start, decide which particular aspects of your mental, emotional, or physical well-being you would want chair yoga to help with. This might be strengthening balance and stability, controlling chronic pain, lowering tension and anxiety, increasing flexibility, or encouraging well-being and relaxation.

**2. Consult with Professionals:** For individualized advice and suggestions, consider speaking with licensed yoga instructors or healthcare providers if you have any particular medical ailments or health concerns. They can provide guidance on appropriate postures, adjustments, and exercises that fit your unique needs and skill level.

**3. Adapt postures as Needed:** Customize your chair yoga practice by adjusting postures to meet your unique physical needs and limits. For instance, you may perform seated variations of common yoga postures like twists, forward bends, and side stretches using a chair if you have restricted knee movement. To maintain comfort and safety, pay attention to your body and modify your practice as necessary.

**4. Emphasize Breath and Mindfulness:** Tailor your chair yoga program to target certain mental and emotional requirements by incorporating breathwork and mindfulness exercises. Mindfulness meditation can improve self-awareness and emotional resilience, while deep breathing exercises can assist relax and soothe the nervous system.

**5. Select Appropriate Practices:** Choose chair yoga poses and routines that are suitable for your level of fitness and expertise. Seek out books, DVDs, or online resources that offer gentle, accessible chair yoga poses that are tailored to the needs of elders or those with limited mobility.

# Overcoming Obstacles and Retaining Drive

**1. Establish Reasonable Expectations:** Acknowledge that chair yoga, like any other type of exercise, requires patience and dedication to improve. For your practice, set attainable yet reasonable goals, and acknowledge minor accomplishments along the way. Be patient with yourself as you overcome obstacles and disappointments, and keep your attention on the process rather than the result.

**2. Find What Motivates You:** Find the things that spur you on to keep practicing chair yoga. Determine what most strongly resonates with you, whether it be the health advantages, the feeling of calm and well-being, or the chance for personal development and self-care, and utilize that motivation to remain dedicated to your practice.

**3. Remain Consistent:** Make consistency a priority in your chair yoga practice by creating a regular practice schedule. Set up time for your practice sessions every day or every week, and consider them to be non-negotiable meetings with yourself. Developing momentum and sustaining enthusiasm over time need consistency.

**4. Find Accountability and Support:** Surround yourself with others who share your passion in chair yoga and who can provide you support. Participate in online forums or social media groups, attend a nearby chair yoga session, or pair up with a friend or relative for accountability and support.

**5. Embrace Variety and Creativity:** Try experimenting with different poses, sequences, and approaches to keep your chair yoga practice interesting and dynamic. Try out several chair yoga methods, such restorative, gentle flow, or chair-based Pilates, to see which suits your body and tastes the best. Keep an open mind to fresh perspectives and methods, and let your practice develop naturally over time.

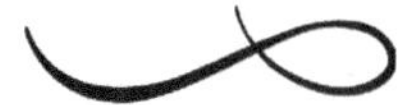

# Chapter Six

# Pain Reduction Exercises and More

This chapter will cover specific exercises that are intended to relieve typical aches and pains that older adults encounter. These soft motions and stretches can ease stiffness, increase range of motion, and enhance general comfort and wellbeing.

# Intended Exercises to Reduce Common Pains and Aches

**1. Neck Rolls:** Take a comfortable seat in your chair, keeping your shoulders loose and your spine straight. Bring your ear close to your shoulder while you gently cock your head to one side. Bring your chin to your chest by slowly rolling your head forward. Then, turn your head to the other side and bring your other ear to your shoulder. Make numerous repetitions of this mild rolling motion while shifting your head from side to side. This exercise facilitates relaxation and increased range of motion by releasing tension in the shoulders and neck.

**2. Shoulder Shrugs:** Keep your arms at your sides while sitting erect in your chair. Take a breath and raise your shoulders to your ears, tensely craning them. Breathe out as you let your shoulders drop back down and fully relax. Release tension and stress from the shoulders and upper back by doing this shoulder shrugging action many times.

**3. Seated Spinal Twist:** Assume a seated position toward the front of the chair, keeping your back straight and your feet level on the ground. For support, place your left hand on the chair's back and your right hand on the outside of your left knee. Breathe in as you extend your back and out as you turn your body slightly to the left and glance over your left shoulder. Feel the mild stretch along the spine as you hold this sitting spinal twist for a few breaths. Continue on the opposite side. This exercise releases stress in the hips and back and enhances spinal mobility.

**4. Sitting Forward Fold:** Place your feet level on the floor and your spine straight as you sit closer to the front of the chair. Breathe in as you extend your back and out as you bend forward from your hips and extend your hands to the floor or your feet. Feel the backs of your legs and spine gently stretch as you let your head drop down your knees. Take a few deep breaths to hold this sitting forward fold, and then gently return to a seated posture. This exercise promotes flexibility and comfort by easing tension in the hamstrings and lower back.

**5. Angle Circles:** Take a comfortable seat and place your feet flat on the ground. Elevate one foot off the floor and start rotating your ankle clockwise and counterclockwise in a circular manner. Feel a light stretch and release in your calves and ankles as you concentrate on moving with control and fluidity. On the other foot, repeat. This exercise lessens stiffness and soreness by increasing ankle mobility and circulation.

*By adding these focused workouts to your regular regimen, you may enhance flexibility, reduce frequent aches and pains, and advance general comfort and wellbeing. Exercise with awareness and mindfulness, paying attention to your body's cues and modifying the poses to fit your unique requirements and capabilities.*

## Methods to Improve Comfort and Mobility

In this part, we'll look at a number of methods created especially to help seniors doing chair yoga feel more mobile and comfortable. Through the use of these mild techniques, people will be able to move more freely and pleasantly in their everyday lives by improving circulation, increasing flexibility, and decreasing stiffness.

**1. Joint Mobilization Exercises**: To improve range of motion and lessen joint stiffness, engage in mild joint mobilization exercises. Shoulder shrugs, ankle rolls, and wrist circles are a few examples of this. To minimize strain or discomfort, move each joint through its entire range of motion while moving slowly and deliberately.

**2. Dynamic Stretching:** To warm up the muscles and get the body ready for activity, incorporate dynamic stretching exercises. This can involve soft motions like torso twists, leg kicks, and arm swings. While you stretch, pay close attention to keeping your motions fluid and smooth. Breathe deeply.

**3. Seated Cat-Cow Stretch:** Place your hands on your knees and sit facing the front of the chair with your feet flat on the ground. Breathe in as you bring your shoulders back, arch your back, and raise your chest toward the ceiling. Tuck your chin into your chest and bring your belly button toward your spine as you exhale and circle your spine. Stretch your spine many times while sitting up straight, using your breath to help release tension and increase range of motion.

## 4. Seated Forward Bend:

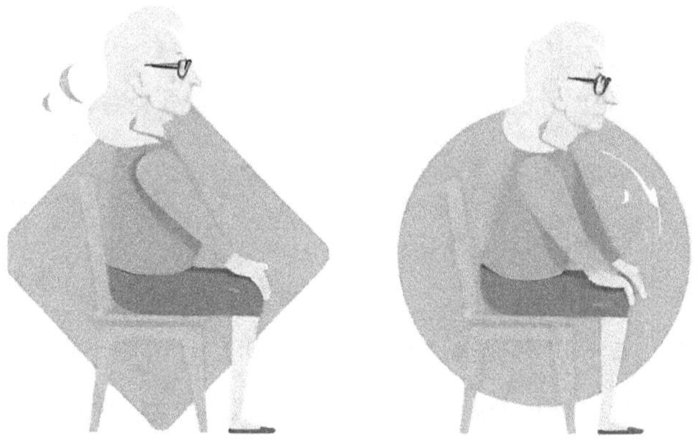

Assume a forward-leaning position, keeping your spine upright and your feet flat on the ground. Breathe in as you extend your back and out as you bend forward from your hips and extend your hands to the floor or your feet. Feel the backs of your legs and spine gently stretch as you let your head drop down your knees. Take a few deep breaths to maintain this sitting forward bend, and then gently return to a seated posture. This stretch encourages comfort and flexibility by easing tension in the hamstrings and lower back.

**5. Incorporate Breathing Techniques:** To help soothe the body and mind, use deep breathing exercises. To engage in diaphragmatic breathing, take a deep inhale through your nose and let your abdomen fill up completely. To fully empty your lungs, exhale softly via your lips while bringing your belly to your spine. Several times over, repeat this deep breathing pattern while paying attention to the feeling of the breath entering and exiting your body.

**6. attentive Movement :** During your chair yoga practice, focus on being attentive to every movement and sensation in your body. To encourage ease and comfort, pay attention to any regions that are tense or uncomfortable and modify your motions accordingly. You may develop a closer relationship with your body and a better understanding of your physical capabilities and limits by engaging in mindful movement.

By using these methods in your chair yoga practice, you may improve mobility, lessen pain, and encourage general health. Keep in mind to move slowly and deliberately, pay attention to your body's cues, and modify the exercises' intensity as necessary to meet your comfort level and specific demands.

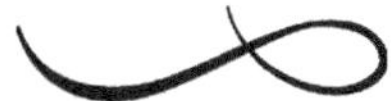

# Chapter Seven

# Nutrient-Key Optimization for Vitality: Seniors Over 60

Keeping up a healthy diet becomes more crucial as we get older to preserve our vigor and general health. A balanced diet high in critical nutrients is crucial for seniors doing chair yoga to maintain their mobility, comfort, and overall health.

Seniors over 60 should prioritize adding nutrient-dense foods, such as fruits, vegetables, whole grains, lean meats, and healthy fats, to their meals. These foods are rich in fiber, vitamins, minerals, and antioxidants, all of which are vital for maintaining general health and lowering the risk of chronic illnesses.

For seniors, calcium and vitamin D are especially crucial since they support bone health and stave off osteoporosis. Together with vitamin D from sources like fatty fish, eggs, and sunshine exposure, including calcium sources like dairy products, leafy greens, and fortified meals can help promote bone strength and mobility.

Omega-3 fatty acids are good for seniors with arthritis or other musculoskeletal problems because they contain anti-inflammatory qualities that can help lessen joint discomfort and stiffness. You can get omega-3 fatty acids in walnuts, flaxseeds, and fatty seafood.

Foods high in antioxidants, such nuts, berries, and dark leafy greens, aid in the fight against oxidative stress and inflammation, two factors that frequently lead to health problems associated with aging. Consuming these meals can promote overall vitality, joint health, and cognitive function.

Finally, for elders to maintain optimal body processes, such as digestion and joint lubrication, they must drink plenty of water. Throughout the day, consuming a sufficient amount of water will assist avoid dehydration and enhance general comfort when doing chair yoga.

Seniors may improve their mobility, comfort, and general well-being by emphasizing a balanced diet full of vital nutrients. This will also help them to get the most out of their chair yoga practice and lead more active and satisfying lives.

# Nutritional Advice for Elderly Chair Yoga Practitioners

Seniors who practice chair yoga might improve their general well-being and comfort level by monitoring their dietary intake. The following dietary advice is intended especially for senior chair yoga practitioners:

**1. Make Protein Your Top Priority:** As people age, seniors require more protein to maintain muscular strength and repair. To promote muscle health and recovery, include lean protein sources like fish, chicken, tofu, beans, and lentils in your meals.

**2. Pay Attention to Whole Foods:** To optimize nutritional advantages, select whole, minimally processed foods wherever feasible. Essential vitamins, minerals, and antioxidants found in whole grains, fruits, vegetables, and lean meats promote general health and wellbeing.

**3. Mindful Eating:** Make conscious meal choices by observing your body's signals of hunger and fullness as well as the flavor, texture, and enjoyment of your food. In addition to preventing overeating, eating mindfully and slowly helps improve digestion.

**4. Remain Hydrated:** Drinking enough water during chair yoga sessions is essential for preserving digestion, joint health, and general comfort. Throughout the day, sip on lots of water and think about including items high in water content, including fruits and vegetables, in your meals and snacks.

**5. Balance Macronutrients:** To maintain energy levels, muscular function, and general vitality, strive for a balanced diet that contains a combination of carbs, protein, and healthy fats. Incorporate lean protein sources, unsaturated fats from foods like avocados, almonds, and olive oil, and complex carbs from whole grains.

**6. Supplement Wisely:** If you have dietary limitations or reside in a location with little sun exposure, you may want to think about adding vitamins or minerals, including vitamin B12 or vitamin D, to your diet to make up for any deficiencies. If you're unsure if supplements are right for you, speak with a medical practitioner.

*Senior chair yoga practitioners may maximize their comfort, wellbeing, and general pleasure of their yoga practice by emphasizing wholesome, nutritional foods and mindful dietary practices. In order for seniors to completely benefit from chair yoga and have active, satisfying lives, they must eat a well-rounded diet that promotes their physical mobility, mental clarity, and emotional well-being.*

# Nutritious Techniques to Increase Senior Chair Yogart's Mobility and Comfort

When it comes to promoting seniors' mobility, comfort, and general well-being during chair yoga sessions, nutrition is crucial. Seniors may increase the advantages of their yoga practice, minimize pain, and maximize their energy levels by using particular dietary measures. The following are some essential tactics to support your chair yoga practice:

**1. Pre-Practice Fuel:** provide your body a healthy lunch or snack that will provide you continuous energy before your chair yoga practice. Choose lean protein sources like yogurt, almonds, or lean meats in addition to complex carbs like whole grains, fruits, and vegetables. These foods include vital nutrients that assist maintain energy levels during your practice and promote muscular performance.

**2. Hydration Hydration is Key:** During chair yoga sessions, maintaining joint lubrication, bolstering muscular performance, and controlling body temperature all depend on adequate hydration. In addition to consuming plenty of water throughout the day, you should think about hydrating drinks like coconut water or herbal tea both before and after your workout. During your yoga practices, being properly hydrated can help avoid weariness, cramps, and discomfort.

**3. Post-session Recovery:** Make sure to give your body the nourishment it needs by replenishing with nutrient-rich meals after your chair yoga session. To aid in muscle healing and refueling, try to eat a combination of carbs and protein within 30 to 60 minutes after your workout. This might be a tiny snack such as a fruit and nut butter piece, a yogurt parfait topped with granola, or a fruit and veggie protein smoothie.

**4. Anti-Inflammatory Foods:** If you suffer from ailments like arthritis or joint pain, including anti-inflammatory foods in your diet to help reduce inflammation and ease suffering. Incorporate foods high in antioxidants and color-rich fruits and vegetables with high omega-3 fatty acid content, such as walnuts, flaxseeds, and fatty salmon. These meals can ease stiffness in your joints, enhance general comfort during your yoga practice, and improve joint health.

**5. Listen to Your Body:** Observe your body's reactions to various meals prior to, during, and following your chair yoga session. Observe how particular meals affect your digestion, energy levels, and general comfort, and modify your diet appropriately. Since each person has different dietary requirements, it's critical to pay attention to your body's cues and make decisions that will best serve your particular health.

*may enhance your chair yoga practice's comfort, mobility, and general enjoyment by including these dietary suggestions into your regimen. Getting the most out of your yoga sessions and improving your general quality of life as a senior practitioner may be achieved by fueling your body with healthy foods, drinking enough water, and supporting post-practice recovery.*

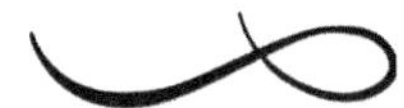

# Chapter Eight

## Feedback and Achievement Reports

We'll feature motivational testimonies and success Stories from older citizens who have benefited greatly from chair yoga in this chapter. These first-hand narratives provide insightful information on the various ways chair yoga may enhance one's physical and mental health as well as general quality of life.

# Motivating Testimonials from Elderly People Who Have Profited from Chair Yoga

**1. Jane's Journey to Mobility:** Jane was reluctant to do chair yoga since she had arthritis, which caused her to have persistent joint discomfort and stiffness. She did, however, decide to give it a go after receiving support from her pals. With persistent work and kind direction from her teacher, Jane's mobility, flexibility, and general comfort improved over time. Chair yoga has become a vital component of her self-care regimen as she feels more empowered and secure in her body.

**2. John's Road to Stress Relief:** During his golden years as a retired businessman, John struggled with stress and anxiety. He looked into chair yoga as a natural, all-encompassing remedy and decided to give it a shot. John found moments of calm and serenity amid life's obstacles by learning to quiet his racing thoughts via daily practice and mindfulness meditation. Chair yoga has grown to be an effective technique for stress relief and improving his general wellbeing.

**3. Mary's Journey to Inner Strength:** Mary was motivated to restore her strength and mobility after undergoing a hip replacement procedure. She added chair yoga to her rehabilitation regimen under the supervision of her physical therapist. Mary gradually regained her strength and confidence with the help of light stretches, strengthening exercises, and mindful breathing methods. She is now stronger, more resilient, and appreciative of chair yoga's therapeutic value in her recuperation process.

**4. Tom's Transformation in Mind and Body:** Tom had always been dubious about yoga, writing it off as "not for him." Nevertheless, in his 60s, he encountered a number of health issues and, on his doctor's advice, he tried chair yoga. To his astonishment, Tom realized early on how beneficial the exercise was. Chair yoga not only helped with his physical ailments but also gave him a much-needed avenue for introspection and stress release. Tom is now a devoted chair yoga advocate who shares his experience to encourage others to discover the life-changing possibilities of the practice.

These endorsements and case studies provide an insight into the significant positive effects chair yoga may have on seniors' life, promoting emotional fortitude, spiritual health, and physical vigor. Every narrative serves as a reminder of the human spirit's tenacity and yoga's transforming potential to inspire and heal people of all ages and abilities.

# Transformative and Healing Personal Journeys

In this section, we go more deeply into the personal stories of seniors who, by practicing chair yoga, went on incredible journeys of self-healing and change. These anecdotes demonstrate the significant positive effects that consistent practice may have on one's general quality of life, mental and physical health, and overall well being.

**1. The retired teacher,** Sarah, had always led an active lifestyle until a string of health setbacks left her feeling defeated and demoralized. This is her story of renewal. She was so exhausted and in constant pain that she started to distance herself from things she used to like. Sarah made the decision to look into alternate methods of treating her symptoms and enhancing her wellbeing since she was in severe need of relief. Sarah developed an inner feeling of calm and fortitude as well as a reconnection with her body under the kind supervision of a chair yoga instructor. She had a fresh feeling of energy and purpose with every breath and movement. Sarah saw a gradual decrease in her discomfort, an upsurge in her vitality, and a renewed appreciation for life's small joys. Chair yoga evolved to become a haven for healing and change as well as a type of exercise.

**2. Michael's Journey to Empowerment:** As a result of injuries he received while serving his country, retired veteran Michael battled PTSD and chronic pain. He struggled to get relief from his symptoms and felt stuck in a cycle of hopelessness and loneliness for many years. Michael looked to chair yoga as a possible therapeutic method because he was determined to take back his life and discover a purpose. Though he was at first dubious, he was shocked to discover that the slow motions and deliberate breathing exercises gave him a sense of peace and stability that he hadn't felt in years. With regular practice and the encouragement of other practitioners, Michael started to develop a fresh sense of empowerment and self-awareness. He found a safe haven in chair yoga, where he could face his inner demons and develop the resilience and elegance to face life's obstacles. Michael still embraces his recovery path today, drawing comfort and strength from chair yoga.

**3. Evelyn's Road to Self-Discovery:** A recent widow, Evelyn struggled with loneliness and sadness following the death of her husband of fifty years. She was having a hard time adjusting to his departure, feeling lost and not sure where to go. Evelyn resorted to chair yoga as a way to nourish her body, mind, and soul in search of comfort and connection. Evelyn regained the sense of belonging and community she had been lacking with the help of her other practitioners and the kind direction of her instructor. She was able to let go of her sadness and welcome the present moment with open arms as a deep sense of acceptance and serenity washed over her with every breath and movement. Evelyn found that chair yoga provided a haven of healing and self-discovery amongst her suffering, which she eventually began to rely on.

*These individual experiences of growth and recovery act as potent reminders of the human spirit's resiliency and its potential for development and rejuvenation even in the face of hardship. Seniors like Sarah, Michael, and Evelyn have discovered a way to self-discovery, empowerment, and healing via chair yoga, demonstrating the transforming power of yoga to heal and uplift the body, mind, and spirit.*

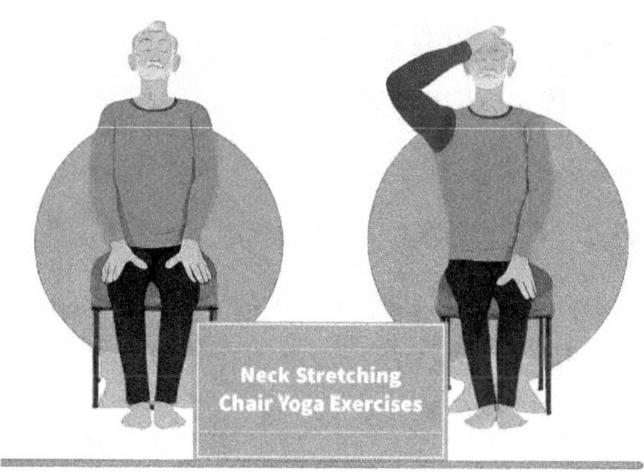
Neck Stretching
Chair Yoga Exercises

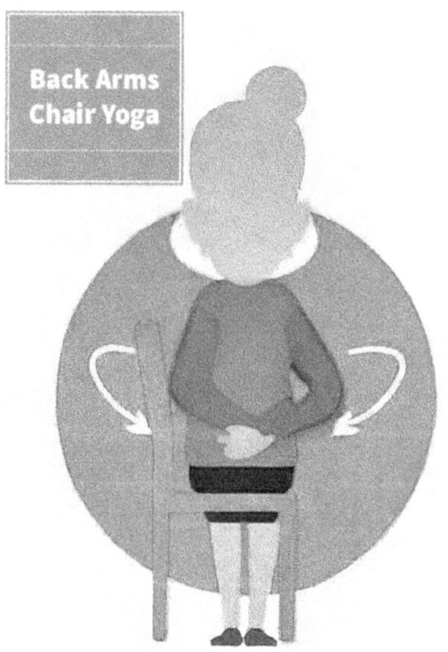
Back Arms
Chair Yoga

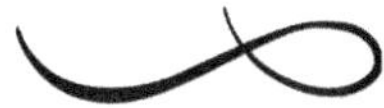

# Chapter Nine

# Experienced Guidance and Resources

In this chapter, you'll find valuable insights and resources from experienced yoga instructors and healthcare professionals, offering guidance to support your chair yoga practice and enhance your overall well-being.

# Tips from Experienced Yoga Instructors and Healthcare Professionals

**1. Correct Alignment and Posture:** Discover the significance of correct alignment in chair yoga poses to minimize risks and enhance advantages. Skilled yoga instructors offer hints and cues to assist you in safely and efficiently aligning your body during practice.

**2. Breathing methods:** During chair yoga classes, learn different breathing methods from yoga instructors and medical specialists to help you relax, decrease stress, and improve awareness. To make your practice more harmonic, learn to connect your breath with your movement.

**3. Adaptations and Modifications:** Learn how to modify chair yoga postures to meet a range of physical restrictions, mobility levels, and skills. Skilled teachers provide innovative ways to make postures approachable and entertaining for all students.

**4. Injury Prevention and Management:** Get professional guidance from medical specialists on preventing injuries and treating them, including information on how to take care of long-term ailments like osteoporosis, arthritis, and joint pain. Discover how to adjust postures and exercises to promote healing and lessen pain.

**5. Progression and Challenge:** Learn how to deepen stretches, boost intensity, and enhance balance and stability as you advance and challenge your chair yoga practice. Skilled teachers offer advice on how to safely advance your practice while acknowledging the limitations of your body.

**6. Mind-Body Connection:** Medical experts underline the value of the mind-body connection when practicing chair yoga, emphasizing the role that mindfulness plays in fostering emotional health and lowering stress levels. Seniors are urged to develop an inner peace and awareness, pay attention to bodily sensations, and concentrate on the here and now.

**7. Community and Support:** Learn how to keep up a regular chair yoga practice by understanding the value of community and support. Learn about the experiences and endorsements of other practitioners, and discover opportunities for networking with like-minded people and enrolling in courses and group sessions.

**8. Additional Information and Resources:** To learn more about chair yoga and related subjects, have access to a carefully chosen collection of suggested books, websites, and learning aids. Investigate other learning and development opportunities to aid in your continuous pursuit of health and wellbeing.

*You may support your chair yoga practice and improve your general quality of life by utilizing the knowledge and skills of seasoned yoga instructors and medical specialists. Their direction will enable you to develop strength, flexibility, balance, and peace of mind on your path to wellbeing, regardless of your level of experience.*

# Locating Chair Yoga Workshops and Classes in Your Region

This section offers helpful advice on where to find chair yoga sessions and courses in your area that are especially designed with seniors in mind. Using these tools can improve your chair yoga practice and help you on your path to better mobility, comfort, and wellbeing, regardless of your level of expertise.

**1. Senior and Community Centers:** For chair yoga courses tailored to the needs of elderly citizens, inquire at your neighborhood community centers, senior centers, or recreation centers. These facilities frequently provide a range of health activities and could regularly have chair yoga classes taught by qualified teachers.

**2. Yoga Studios:** Seniors and anyone with restricted mobility can take advantage of the chair yoga courses that many yoga studios provide. Look into local studios and find out what classes they offer. Make sure the studios can adjust and modify the lesson to meet your needs.

**3. Medical Facilities and Rehab institutions:** As an adjunct to their treatment services or wellness efforts, hospitals, clinics, and rehabilitation institutions may provide chair yoga programs. Healthcare specialists with training in modifying yoga poses for people with different health conditions frequently lead these sessions.

**4. Virtual Platforms and Online Resources:** Look into virtual platforms and online resources that provide senior chair yoga courses and workshops. You may be able to practice in the comfort of your own home by using websites, apps, and social media platforms to have access to guided sessions taught by qualified teachers.

**5. Community Events and Workshops:** Look for opportunities to practice chair yoga, such as workshops, health fairs, and community events. These gatherings offer chances to meet local teachers, pick up new skills, and experiment with various chair yoga practices.

**6. Word of Mouth and Referrals :** Speak with seniors, friends, or family members who may know someone who has taken chair yoga sessions locally. They may assist you in selecting the ideal course or teacher for your requirements by offering suggestions, analysis, and firsthand knowledge.

*You may locate chair yoga classes and workshops in your region by looking through these options. By doing so, you'll have access to helpful tools and assistance that will improve your practice and advance your general wellbeing. Seniors looking to include chair yoga into their everyday life have a plethora of alternatives at their disposal, whether they choose virtual or in-person sessions.*

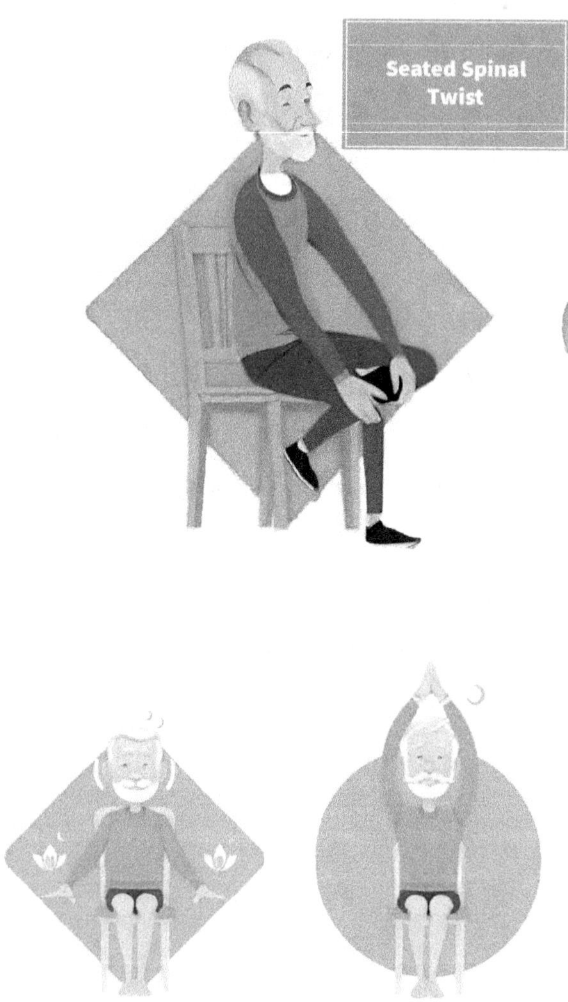
Seated Spinal
Twist

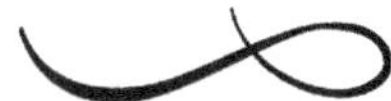

# Chapter Ten

## 30-Day Success Challenge

This chapter offers a comprehensive 30-day success plan that has been painstakingly designed to help seniors get started with chair yoga. Every stage is thoughtfully crafted to guarantee a steady and fulfilling advancement, promoting not only physical enhancement but also mental clarity and emotional stability.

# First Week: Fundamentals and Orientation

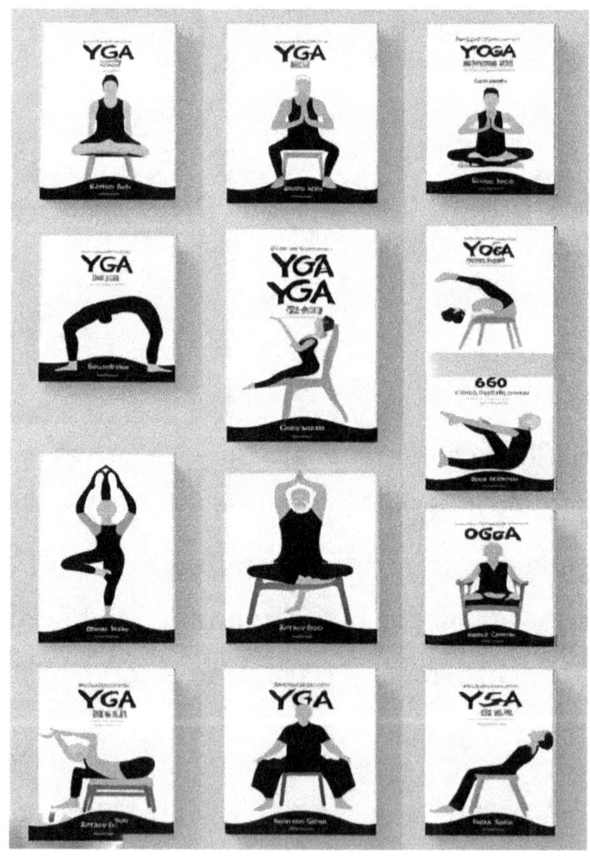

**Days 1-3: Introduction to Chair Yoga -** To start, dedicate 10 to 15 minutes a day to learning the fundamentals of chair yoga.

- Take a seat comfortably in a solid chair and concentrate on keeping your posture straight and your feet planted firmly.

- Engage in deep breathing techniques to promote awareness and relaxation. Breathe in deeply from your nose and out completely through your mouth.

- Learn basic poses with an emphasis on alignment and gentle movements, such as the Seated Mountain Pose, Seated Forward Fold, and Seated Twist.

**Days 4–7: Forming a Schedule**

- Find a regular time and place for your chair yoga sessions, then gradually extend your practice duration to 15 to 20 minutes each day.

- Try varying your hours of sleep to find out when you are most alert and concentrated—in the morning, in the afternoon, or at night.

- To keep yourself motivated and dedicated to your routine, choose an aim for your practice, such as increasing mobility, decreasing stress, or improving flexibility.

# Week 2: Developing Stability and Strength

## - Days 8–14: Exercises to Develop Strength

- Start adding strength-training poses to your chair yoga practice, emphasizing body stabilization and core muscular engagement.

- Try positions like Chair Warrior, Chair Cat-Cow, and Chair Bridge to strengthen and stabilize your body while focusing on your key muscle groups.

- As you practice, gradually extend its length and intensity, pushing yourself to stay in good alignment and be mindful of your breath.

## - Days 15–21: Stability and Balance

- Set aside time each day to work on proprioception and coordination via balancing postures and exercises.

- Begin with easy balancing exercises like sitting with one foot elevated off the ground or using a chair's back as support.

- Advance to increasingly difficult postures, such as Half Moon, Eagle, and Tree Pose, utilizing the chair for support as necessary.

# Week 3: Adaptability and Calmness

**Days 22–24: Mild Stretching –** To increase flexibility and relieve tension in the muscles and joints, concentrate on mild stretching and mobility exercises.

- Incorporate dynamic exercises to warm up the body and get ready for deeper stretches, such as spinal twists, shoulder rolls, and neck rolls. Examine sitting stretches for your neck, shoulders, back, hips, and legs while paying attention to your body's limits and moving thoughtfully.

**Days 25–28: Relieving Stress and Rejuvenation**

- Set aside time each day to practice relaxation methods that help you feel less stressed and more at peace with yourself.

- To calm the mind and calm the nervous system, engage in gradual muscle relaxation, guided visualization, and deep breathing techniques.

- Develop an attitude of thankfulness and appreciation for the here and now, realizing the positive effects of your chair yoga practice on your general health.

# Week 4: Integration and Reflection

**Day 29: Integration Session** - Incorporate aspects of the practices from the previous weeks into a thorough chair yoga practice that flows naturally from one posture to the next.

- Finding a balance between effort and ease, concentrate on fluidity, breath awareness, and mindfulness as you go through the sequence.

- Take pauses when necessary, pay attention to your body's cues, and modify the level of difficulty of your practice to fit your comfort and energy levels.

## - Day 30: Contemplation and Festivity

- Examine your chair yoga experience over the last 30 days, noting your accomplishments and the obstacles you've surmounted.

- Acknowledge your accomplishments, no matter how minor, and show your thanks for the chance to learn about chair yoga and its advantages.

- Make plans for your yoga practice's continued development and discovery, understanding that it's a never-ending journey with endless opportunities.

Seniors who devote themselves fully to this complete 30-day success plan can see noticeable gains in their general well-being, strength, mobility, and balance. Every phase in the chair yoga journey is designed to facilitate sustained growth and progressive advancement, so you can expect a life-changing and fulfilling experience that lasts far beyond the 30-day period.

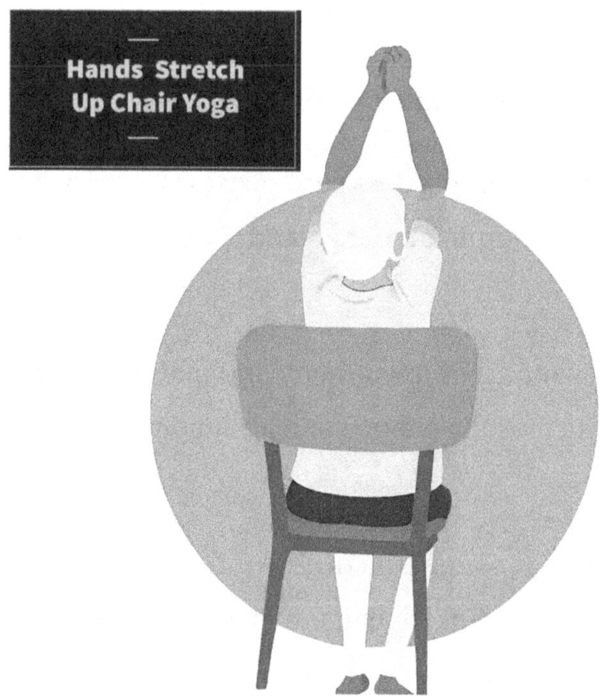

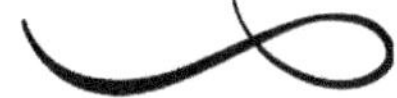

# Conclusion

As we come to the end of our investigation into chair yoga for seniors over 60, it is important to consider the life-changing potential of this practice. We've covered a wide range of chair yoga advantages in this book, from increased flexibility and strength to better sleep and stress reduction.

For seniors looking to retain their flexibility, stay active, and enhance their general well-being, chair yoga provides a mild yet effective approach. We've found that by modifying classic yoga postures for the sitting posture, people of all ages and skill levels may benefit from this practice.

In addition to its physical advantages, chair yoga offers a route towards mental and emotional well-being. Deep breathing exercises, relaxation methods, and mindfulness meditation have taught us how to create inner calm, lower stress levels, and develop appreciation for the now.

It's important to put self-care first and adopt habits that feed our bodies, brains, and spirits as we navigate our golden years. A more comprehensive approach to wellbeing is provided by chair yoga, which encourages us to live more completely in the present and establish deeper connections with ourselves.

I urge everyone, regardless of experience level, to keep learning about and implementing chair yoga into their everyday routine. Accept the path to wellness with an open mind and a readiness to change, develop, and learn as you go.

I hope this book will be a source of inspiration and guidance for you as you embark on your chair yoga adventure, enabling you to maintain a healthy, balanced, and joyful life long into your golden years. Recall that the journey to wellbeing is an ongoing practice of self-care and self-discovery rather than a final destination. Accept the voyage, and may it be filled with plenty of happiness, health, and tranquility.

## Bonus Resources  Chair Yoga for Seniors

## Scan the Qr code Below

# Appendix

## Practice Sequences and an Illustrated Pose Guide

A thorough collection of illustrated chair yoga postures and practice sequences to assist you on your path to wellbeing may be found in this appendix. To guarantee correct alignment and execution, each posture comes with comprehensive instructions and visual aids.

## First Section: Detailed Pose Guide

- Mountain Pose (seated), Forward Fold (seated), Twist (seated), Chair Warrior (seated), Chair Cat-Cow (seated), Chair Bridge (seated), and Seated Knee Lifts

- Extended Legs While Seated

- Chair-Sided Kicks

The following poses may be done using a chair: Tree Pose, Eagle Pose, Dancer Pose.

## Practice Sequences: Section 2

**- Gentle Warm-Up Sequence:** A set of soft stretches and motions to increase flexibility and get the body ready for practice.

**- Strength-Building Sequence:** This set of postures aims to strengthen the muscles in the upper body, lower body, and core.

**- Balance and Stability Sequence:** A set of exercises and positions for balance that enhance proprioception, coordination, and stability.

**- Relaxation and Stress Relief Sequence:** A series of relaxation methods to encourage stress reduction and rejuvenation, such as progressive muscle relaxation, guided imagery, and deep breathing exercises.

*Every exercise routine is intended to be both flexible and accessible to people of all skill levels. You'll discover a range of positions and sequences to suit your individual requirements and goals, regardless of your level of expertise.*

Preston Arias

*Dear Reader,*

*I'm reaching out to express my gratitude for your support in acquiring "Chair Yoga for Seniors Over 60." Your interest in exploring the transformative practice of chair yoga means a great deal to me.*

*As an author, nothing brings me more joy than knowing my work positively impacts readers' lives. Could I kindly ask for a moment of your time to share your thoughts and experiences by leaving a positive review for the book?*

*Your review not only provides valuable feedback but also helps guide other potential readers. Whether you found the book informative, inspiring, or thought-provoking, your honest review will be invaluable.*

*Thank you for contributing to a community seeking healthier, happier lives through chair yoga. Your positive review will make a significant difference.*

*With warm regards,*

*[Preston Arias]*

# Index

*Preston Arias*

## E



## F



## G



## I

www.ingramcontent.com/pod-product-compliance
Lightning Source LLC
Chambersburg PA
CBHW050928260726
48660CB00001B/454